Fighting
Covid
Naturally

G SAMBI

Fighting Covid Naturally

A life-changing herb that does wonders!

G SAMBI

First edition

Published by

Jolly Books Publishing House

By arrangements with

Kindle Direct Publishing

Please visit: jollybookspublishing.com or jollybookspublishing.co.uk

The human body is a concoction of five elements: earth, water, air, fire and ether. Physical health, mental health, emotional well-being and happiness can be restored by simply getting the balance of these elements right.

- G Sambi

CONTENTS

ACKNOWLEDGMENTS   I

CHAPTER 1: INTRODUCTION   1

CHAPTER 2: CAUSE OF CORONAVIRUS   7

CHAPTER 3: SYMPTOMS OF COVID-19   11

CHAPTER 4: DISCOVERY OF THE WONDER HERB   17

CHAPTER 5: DEFEATING COVID-19 AGAIN   46

CHAPTER 6: THE WONDER HERB DISCUSSED   61

CHAPTER 7: AMAZING RESULTS RE-CONFIRMED   73

CHAPTER 8: PROPER ADMINISTRATION OF THE HERB 78

CHAPTER 9: COVID AND MENTAL HEALTH   82

ABOUT THE AUTHOR   93

Fighting Covid Naturally

ACKNOWLEDGMENTS

I would first like to thank the divine power that pervades in us all, which has lovingly guided and protected me.

My special thanks to my spiritual master, who introduced me to the mysteries of the beyond. That has been one of the most significant moments of my life, which has opened up spiritual avenues that were previously incomprehensible. To him, I will always remain deeply indebted.

Additionally, I would like to thank all the philosophers, naturopaths, homeopaths and medical researchers who have contributed throughout different ages to the study and development of health and eradication of maladies.

This book would not have been possible without the love and support of my wife and nearly 3-year-old daughter, who sacrificed our much-cherished family time to support me in completing this book all through to its publication. I am immensely grateful to them.

CHAPTER 1

Introduction

One cannot fully understand health and well-being without understanding the composition of the human body. It is the imbalance in the human body's design that leads to all illnesses. Therefore optimum health is achieved by understanding the subtle balance of the body to avoid complications altogether or attrition its effects.

Covid-19 and its variants are no exception to balancing the elements to fight back the illness. The virus is an external agent that creates an imbalance within the body for its survival and regeneration. This imbalance simply needs to be addressed, and the virus can then not thrive.

The concept is simple, yet dealing with a completely new and unknown external agent, i.e. the virus that has created the imbalance, is not easy. Whether it is modern science or complementary medicine, or ancient wisdom, the health practitioner or the naturopath aims to find an external agent, i.e. a remedy that would create a balancing environment in the body to counter the imbalance created by the virus. In the long term, that would also boost the body's natural balancing mechanism to fight back and restore harmony.

Complex structure of the elements and the microbiome

The human body is comprised of five main elements. These are the earth, water, fire, air and ether. These five elements have an effect on the microbiome within us. Consequentially, the microbiome creates an environment where it may impact us positively or negatively.

If the body is well balanced with the five elements,

we have a healthy microbiome and a healthy body.

If an external micro-organism such as Covid comes into contact with the human body, it attaches itself to it, and in Covid's case, it is through the lungs. It then begins to thrive there, creating the illness. To hinder such an unwanted agent's growth, we need the assistance of the elements to attack the virus and rehabilitate the body.

The Covid illness' impact varies on an individual to individual basis as it depends on the requisite synergy between the five elements and the microbiome. Such synergy is different in each individual due to the body's varying elemental composition resulting in the microbiome's different complex structure that impacts the immune health.

Therefore, infants are more readily able to fight Covid due to their elemental composition and microbiome being in a good state. With age, poor diet, bad habits, and existing medical conditions, the body's fighting mechanism has a predisposition to fight a new virus.

The Covid saga

The advent of coronavirus has taken the entire world into its grasp. Economies have significantly suffered, jobs have been lost, and many more jobs put to scrutiny.

We have seen our freedom curtailed. People have been distanced from their loved ones due to this newly found virus (or recently mutated virus) that has brought havoc into our lives.

Many vaccinations have come out lately to deal with this virus, and as this virus mutates further, different strains have emerged. The vaccines will hopefully be altered to deal with the new strains in time.

While vaccines have been a product of modern science, it has been accepted in general that they are a friend rather than a foe of humanity. The reason is that vaccines, generally speaking, do not go against the body's natural processes. Therefore, the author is not at all averse to the idea of vaccination.

There are many sceptics of the new vaccines given that it has not been observed for a long time before being made available publicly. The vaccines that exist are proving to be somewhat quite good but not 100% effective to deal with coronavirus. Some have shown efficacy of more than 80% for the original covid 19.

Even if one is vaccinated, they can still be infected and show symptoms. However, research does point out that the severity of the symptoms is considerably reduced in most vaccinated individuals.

This book is written so that one may benefit in their fight against dealing with coronavirus symptoms. The author found significant and immediate results with the use of this herb to fight his Covid illness. The herb showed drastic improvement. Others tested positive on coronavirus and displayed severe illness also used this herb and called it "amazing".

The proper use of this inexpensive herb has had some very positive feedback, and the spontaneous relief from coronavirus symptoms was quite miraculous. Therefore, it is hoped that the reader and their loved ones would benefit from this book in the unlikely event they display the unwanted signs of Covid 19 and get confined to their homes.

CHAPTER 2

Cause of coronavirus

A coronavirus is a form of a virus that has taken humanity into its grips. The new mutation is called COVID 19, which is the cause of the 2019-2021 pandemic. Its technical term is severe acute respiratory syndrome coronavirus two or its acronym SARS-Cov-2.

There has been a lot of debate as to how this virus got into the human chain. There have been many theories that have circulated in the news channels regarding its origination. Some speculate that it is a consequence of a laboratory test, while others say it is due to the human consuming bats or snakes. Whatever the speculation may be, one thing is for sure that viruses are part of the ecosystem, and

Covid 19 has become part of the human chain. A problem has been created, and like any other problem, humanity is going to overcome it.

One must realize that virus infections have come in the past, but they were not then part of human life. The condition created by the infection with the new virus creates an imbalance in the human body, resulting in abnormity. The abnormality is displayed by way of illness and symptoms. That is the body's natural reaction in dealing with this new problem, i.e. imbalance and telling us that something is not right

It has now been widely accepted that an infected person can infect others not by touch but through the air, the infected person exhales. As its name suggests, i.e. severe acute respiratory syndrome coronavirus 2 (SARS-Cov-2), it is a respiratory illness, and it's airborne. This means it gets spread through the air and in particular through the water droplets coming out from within the infected person's respiratory tract that carries the virus and, if inhaled by others, infects those as well.

Once the person gets infected, then depending on their immunity, how balanced their body is regarding the five elements and the microbiome, this newly infected person may either have no symptoms whatsoever or mild symptoms or very severe symptoms.

It has been noted that many people with previously known medical conditions or people of old age are more susceptible to this virus. However, many reports have shown that reasonably healthy people or very young people or children have had fatality as well upon being infected by this virus.

It is a very new thing for our present generation, so only with time and more studies will modern scientists know more about this virus. The scientists have done a brilliant job by finding vaccinations that will help tackle this new virus. However, with the new strains of the virus on the scene, vaccines will require a review and update very soon.

The people who may still get infected with severe symptoms despite being inoculated or those deciding not to get vaccinated, or those still waiting to get vaccinated, all combined still does make a large number. Such individuals, if infected, may or may not display symptoms. Hence, the fight against Covid 19 is far from over.

While this new virus's origination in the human chain may still be a mystery, its cause resulting in infection to others is now pretty much undisputed.

Albeit the exhaled air carries the virus, making it airborne, the water droplets within the exhaled air can also land on surfaces. If such contaminated surface is touched and those unwashed and non-sanitized hands then touch the eyes, mouth or nose, it can infect the person.

Therefore, whilst masks may help reduce the infection rate, a face shield covering the eyes is also helpful if one wants to decrease the chances of infection.

CHAPTER 3

Symptoms of Covid-19

A symptom is a body's reaction to deal with the illness in the best possible way available to the human frame.

A symptom is a sign of the body fighting back. Whether the body is winning or losing or barely managing determines the severity of the symptom. Therefore, before the infection, the body's state is crucial because if the body is not healthy and balanced, its fight against the virus may be impacted more than others.

A healthy body will have all its functions working correctly, would be well-balanced and well-nourished with no deficiency of any vitamin or mineral. We see that a child who generally may be born healthy may, with time, get deficient in nutrients resulting in certain parts of the body not getting the nutrients it needs as a fuel to carry out its functions.

The human body is like a piece of complete machinery, and if one part of the machine becomes damaged, then although the machine may continue to work, it may not work as efficiently. With time, if the defective part of the machine is not taken care of, then other parts of the machinery may start getting impacted or may have to work more to compensate due to the damaged part not working or inadequately working.

So just like a piece of damaged machinery causing further damage, if a person already has a pre-medical condition, then the chances are that such person may have a disadvantage to deal with Covid 19.

The root cause lies in imbalance and not a pre-medical condition. The latter is only a consequence of the former.

It is well accepted by the scientific community that people with a pre-medical condition are more susceptible to the virus. Still, there have also been many instances where reasonably healthy people have gone through severe symptoms and even fatality.

Such a generally healthy category of persons who display severe symptoms that needs hospitalization may have an imbalanced constitution due to age, bad habits or some undetected or unnoticeable nutritional deficiency or deficiencies or some emotional condition. That has an impact on one's microbiome, which may look insignificant. Although that may seem ordinary, it does affect the human body.

Humans are like highly complex machinery involving several trillions of micro-organisms for our day to day functions. Minerals and vitamins result in a lot of biochemical reactions, and so to pinpoint the exact specific reason why the severity of symptom varies can sometimes cannot be generalized

Accordingly, a Covid 19 infected person's symptoms will vary from individual to individual, but the cause remains the same, i.e. getting infected primarily through the respiratory system.

Many articles and news channels have reported the symptoms of the virus. They go from being asymptomatic to having fever, breathlessness, shivering, body aches, loss of sense of smell, loss of taste, feeling cold, fatigued, constant coughing etc.

Depending on the country one is based, one should follow the laws and the guidelines set by their respective government, the medical profession and seek medical assistance as per the advice available.

It has been reported around the world that many can deal with the symptoms of the virus at home, and only a small percentage will require hospitalization. However, the logistical problem encountered was that the hospitals would be overwhelmed if that small percentage became infected suddenly. That would mean that the hospitals may not be able to care for all the patients needing hospitalization or requiring medical attention.

The other problem the world faced was that it was unprepared. That was due to the virus' sudden spread.

There were not enough personal protective equipment, sanitization gels, anti-viral gels, masks etc., to deal with this new virus. Also, the virus being new to the scientific community, the true nature of the virus required thorough research to fully understand its nature, remedies, effectiveness, seriousness and impact of this new virus upon humans. Given the time that has lapsed in dealing with this virus, the scientific community and people now understand it more. But still, as of now, it remains not fully understood. The virus produces different reactions in different individuals. The scientific community needs more time to understand the virus and its mutated strains fully.

The herb discussed in the later chapters has shown promising signs to considerably reduce the symptoms of Covid 19, giving the much-needed relief to the sufferer.

CHAPTER 4

Discovery of the wonder herb

My experience with coronavirus has been unique compared to the scientific consensus available at the appropriate time.

It was the end of December 2019, and I, being based in the UK like many others, was to break for the one week plus holiday as offices usually are closed for the last week of the year for Christmas and new year.

Covid 19 was not in the British local news back then. Brits, like the majority of the world, had no clue at that time what is to become known soon.

I cannot remember the precise date, but it was the last two weeks of 2019 when I started to have a sore throat. At the time, I did not think much of it as the sore throat, from my experience in dealing with infections, seemed like a typical infection and a possible sign of fever to follow.

With my previous experiences in dealing with fever and infection generally, I knew that something more severe is to happen in the form of high fever. It was just my body giving me signs of high fever to follow without me having any inclination of the severity of the illness or the type of infection, i.e. bacterial or viral.

Luckily my wife and daughter were travelling abroad during the Christmas break for a family wedding just after the new year. I could not go due to offices re-opening after the new year. So I was all alone in the house during my first Covid infection.

My throat's soreness increased considerably within no time, and even swallowing my saliva caused immense pain in my throat. It was okay for me to speak, although it was uncomfortable to do so, and anything I drank resulted in tremendous pain.

I did not experience any persistent cough, as reported later in February/March 2020. Therefore, I had no clue that it was a new viral infection not experienced by my body before.

As anticipated, I started getting a fever in or around the last week of December 2019. Given that there were no talks about the virus in the United Kingdom, and nobody from the general population had heard about this new virus in the United Kingdom, I began taking it as an infection like encountered many times before. I, therefore, did not think much about it other than to consider it as a common bacterial infection starting with sore throat leading to fever taking its full course before recovery.

Therefore, I was not surprised when I started to get a fever, and then a high fever followed soon. Within no time, I had extreme aches all through the body with extreme fatigue. The aches and fatigue were so intense that I preferred not to move around in the bed, let alone get out of bed to eat something.

My hunger had also nearly gone, or shall I say, taken over by the extreme body ache, tiredness and fever due to the illness. I, therefore, did not feel like eating anyway.

I had experienced a severe sore throat in the past, many years back as part of an infection followed by fever. But the body ache I had this time was simply never experienced before in my 37 years of experience.

Whilst my body temperature was very high, and I was sweating, I was also shivering and feeling extremely cold despite the central heating being on to the full. I had to switch on another portable heater in my bedroom to raise the temperature of the room. It was like a sauna, but I was still shivering despite being wrapped up in a chunky fleece jacket with a duvet on me to no avail.

I simply did not have the energy to chew something, which would not only cause pain in my throat while swallowing, but also the hunger pangs had anyways gone. The body ache and fatigue didn't let me feel comfortable enough to get up and spend the little energy I had on eating. I have done intermittent fasting, so I was not too concerned about not eating for many hours at a stretch. As I was mostly in bed, the demand my body was making for food had also reduced.

I infrequently nibbled to keep the body going and give it fuel to fight back, but that was all. The other reason I had forced myself to eat was to enable me to take some medication afterwards to ease the symptoms.

I am very pro-nature, and I heavily rely on natural-based supplements to heal as naturally as possible. But I am also not averse to taking medicines if I feel that things are not getting back under control or causing me discomfort beyond what is normal for me to function.

Herbs, vitamins and minerals I used to fight my illness

As an ardent (yet realistic) believer and follower of natural healing, I started first by taking natural-based supplements and herbs to tackle the problem when I began to display symptoms.

I take vitamin C regularly, which is well known to boost the immune system. Vitamin C is a water-soluble vitamin, and hence any excess gets drained out of our system through natural processes. That does not mean one should take excessive amounts of vitamin C as it will put a burden on the organs that are draining the excess vitamin C regularly if one is supplementing heavily on it. Therefore moderation is vital when taking such supplements, even if they are naturally based.

I usually take 500 mg of vitamin C with bioflavonoids almost daily. The bioflavonoids make it easier for the body to absorb. Under normal circumstances, I sometimes miss the daily dosage of vitamin C supplement, either just by chance and sometimes on purpose. I do this so that the body does not develop any sensitivity or get used to it or dependent on it to such an extent that it does not make any effort to get vitamin C from the everyday food I consume.

At times I also take 1000 mg of vitamin C supplement with bioflavonoids.

Having an occasional intermittent break from regular supplementation prevents the body getting used to the easy nutritional feed it gets.

Just like any life form that thrives more and becomes more robust when faced with challenges, the human body also thrives more and becomes stronger when it is put to challenge. So it is essential not to make the body dependent on supplementation unless medically advised otherwise.

A normal functioning healthy body should not be made entirely dependent on vitamins and minerals supplementation to such an extent that it stops working efficiently in digesting and absorbing nutrients from regular food that requires a little more effort. Hence, an occasional break from supplements for a day or two, or possibly up to a week, in my opinion, is beneficial for optimum health.

Giving too long breaks is not something I would recommend unless one's diet is reasonably well balanced and coming from an organic source.

As I took vitamin C more or less regularly, my immune system was not hampered due to a lack of this vitamin. It is widely known that vitamin C is good for the immune system, and one is to have reasonably good levels to fight the virus or, generally speaking, for good health.

The other widely discussed vitamin for good immunity is vitamin D. Vitamin D3 form is the one which is considered more beneficial than any other form of vitamin D supplements.

Vitamin D is a fat-soluble vitamin, and hence it needs to be taken with food containing some sort of fat to make it absorbable in the body. With the advent of the new virus, vitamin D and vitamin C supplements had been mentioned in the news quite a bit. So these two vitamins should not come as a surprise for somebody trying to boost the immune system, generally speaking.

The dosage of vitamin D, however, is a debatable issue. Whilst some may say 400 international units (IU) a day may be sufficient, for some, even 4000 international units a day may be slightly less than adequate for optimum health. Therefore, getting your blood work done for vitamin D helps to understand where one stands as far as vitamin D is concerned. Based on that, you can increase or decrease your dosage unless medically advised not to do so.

My requirement for vitamin D levels is relatively high, and I usually take 50,000 international units in tablet form every 10-14 days for maintaining optimum levels of this vitamin in my body. That may seem a very high dosage for people who have not looked more into this vitamin or those who may not require it in such a high amount.

Vitamin D's requirement depends on various factors such as skin colour, genetic disposition, absorption issues, and the amount of exposure to sunlight. One's geographical location also has a significant impact on the quality of sunlight one gets. Therefore, regular biannual bloodwork helps monitor the levels of vitamin D instead of taking a conjectural approach.

Furthermore, Vitamin D gets stored in the body, and excess can be toxic, so getting bloodwork done is quite helpful.

Like vitamin C, I regularly supplemented and monitored Vitamin D. Consequentially, my immune system did not take a hit because of the vitamin D levels.

Apart from these two commonly talked about

vitamins for the immune system that has done good rounds recently due to the Covid 19 outbreak, there are many other supplements, vitamins and minerals that work to help with immunity which I took and discuss here.

Magnesium is a mineral needed for the body to make optimum use of vitamin D. Magnesium is also required for muscles and bones. Therefore, one should keep track of the magnesium level for immunity due to its co-relation with vitamin D that impacts immunity and its positive effects on muscles.

I usually take 400 mg of the ionic form of magnesium orally, which is not only natural but one of the most bioavailable forms available. I also use magnesium oil at times on the skin, which is quite readily absorbed by the body.

I was not concerned about my magnesium levels at the time of illness as I was biannually getting my bloodwork done to track this mineral.

It meant that during my Covid 19 illness at December end of 2019, it was not something that I had to worry about to boost my immune system. However, I did continue to take vitamin C, vitamin D, and magnesium during my Covid infection.

Also, when taking vitamin D, one should consider taking vitamin K2 as they work in synergy. Although Vitamin K2 may not be the first few vitamins that come to mind for immunity, it is essential to look into it because of its interaction with vitamin D.

I take vitamin K from a natural based supplement. It is vitamin K2 which works more than any other form of vitamin K.

As I was taking vitamin K as part of my healthy diet, there was no compromise on my immunity due to my body's lack of this vitamin.

As stated before, I continued to take vitamin D, vitamin C, vitamin K and magnesium as usual, even during my Covid illness.

Given that the virus was unknown at that time in the

UK, I had to consider it a fever caused by some infection. I have had a very severe sore throat and a lot of pain in the past, but that was attributable to a bacterial infection.

Garlic is quite good to deal with fever and fighting infection. My standard immediate step to tackle fever or initial symptoms of fever is to take garlic. Garlic clove should be taken raw if possible. To avoid its strong taste, I quickly crush it with my side teeth until it's turned into paste-like in my mouth. I do not savour it and instead, simply gulp it down with 1 pint of water.

Garlic is more helpful if taken raw. When we cut the garlic or crush it outside the mouth, it does lose some of its properties that are beneficial for healing the body. So when I take garlic, I take one or two cloves crushed between my teeth without savouring the taste and rolling it in my mouth or under the tongue and quickly drinking a glass or two full of water.

In naturopathy, one is asked to drink a lot of water when taking garlic in the raw form. Therefore one big glass of water or two big water glasses should be taken when consuming raw garlic.

In naturopathy, cooked garlic, externally crushed garlic, and cut garlic is not the best way to take it when consuming for its healing properties and fever-reducing or infection-fighting properties.

In addition to taking raw garlic, I also took Allicin capsules. Allicin is an ingredient in garlic that the scientific community considers to be the one that gives garlic its health benefits. From the internet search of finding the proper supplementation, I understood that the process of extracting Allicin is crucial as it gets destroyed very quickly. Therefore, one should choose a supplement where Allicin could be found, and extracted through a technology that preserves its effectiveness.

Whether Allicin supplement is an advertisement gimmick or scientifically proven to be far better than garlic capsules is not something I can confirm. However, from my limited use of Allicin supplements generally, it seemed to work for the overall health benefit I usually get from taking raw garlic. I take raw garlic occasionally to maintain decent cholesterol levels, apart from specific occasions to fight fever or infection.

Colloidal silver is also quite effective in fighting bacterial and viral infections. I was taking one tablespoon at the start of my illness. I also gargled with it but did not have any improvement from its use.

Indian basil or tulsi is a herb that is also considered in naturopathy as very effective in dealing with fever and is also considered anti-viral and anti-bacterial. I usually keep dried powder of this herb in my house for general health, and I do take it occasionally but not regularly. To fight this illness, which was unknown in Britain at that time, I took half a teaspoon of dried powdered tulsi herb or Indian basil every day to help in quick healing. I took it with water.

Neem, also known as Azadirachta Indica, is also considered a very important herb for healing purposes. It is suitable for reducing fever and has anti-bacterial and anti-viral properties, which are highly praised in Ayurveda. Neem is exceedingly bitter to taste. As I have a sweet tooth, I generally use neem to balance my sugar intake. I have got used to the taste, so I take powdered form with water for general health.

I took one teaspoon of powdered neem herb with water almost daily to fight the fever and the infection.

Although I took the powdered form, capsules for both tulsi and neem are available in the market. If one is taking the powdered form, then one must bear in mind that neem is very unpleasant in taste due to its extreme bitterness. So one is better off taking its capsule form instead of powdered form for good health rather than struggle with it. Capsules will give the majority of its benefit, although, in Ayurveda, even taste plays a role in getting the full health benefits.

Whilst turmeric is anti-inflammatory, I did not take this herb until the very end of my Covid illness.

Medicines I took to fight my then-unknown illness

The arsenal of herbs, vitamins and minerals I was taking was good to fight minor health issues and boost the immune system generally.

In the case of my Covid infection of end December 2019, I did not see anything discussed above having any significant impact on improving my condition. That does not mean that it was of no use. It may have helped to keep my health from getting entirely out of control. The herb that worked instantaneously has not been discussed above as it was only later that I found it to have a very positive impact.

As far as medication is concerned, it was probably the second day I started taking it when the soreness in the throat had started to increase quite a bit, followed by fever and body ache.

I knew that high fever was to follow, and it was going to be severe. So I started taking two tablets of 500 mg paracetamol every four hours and two tablets of 200 mg of ibuprofen every four hours alternating so that every two hours, I was taking some form of medication. Soon or within a day, I was encountering severe body ache and fever.

For the avoidance of any doubt, I did not exceed or take any excess of the medication no matter how bad my symptoms were at that time. An overdose will put unwanted stress on the organs and so can be counterproductive.

Despite taking all the herbal supplements and medication on the side, the symptoms just seemed to get worse.

I soon realized that this was not any normal fever or typical infection I had ever encountered. The body ache and fatigue I had was something I never experienced ever in my lifetime. Even coming downstairs from my bedroom on the first floor to the kitchen, which was on the ground floor, was a mission in itself. However, I had to make this effort to get water and eat a little bit before taking the medicines.

It would be the second day of my very severe illness to include a very sore throat, that I decided to take some antibiotics. I am not very prompt when taking antibiotics; I only take them as a last resort when all other medications have failed.

Although antibiotics do work, they do create havoc in the microbiome within the body. That is not good in the long run, and so all efforts should be made to re-balance the microbiome by taking probiotics and prebiotics.

I had many previous years ago experienced severe sore throat like this one, followed by fever. On all such occasions, it was a bacterial infection, and antibiotics did work quite well to deal with it.

There was some antibiotic in my house as my mother-in-law had left hers behind. I started to take the antibiotic called Ciprofloxacin on my second day of severe illness, hoping for an improvement.

At this time, the sore throat had already been continuing for about a week. Usually, one sees improvement with antibiotics within hours if dealing with a bacterial infection. I was not showing any signs of improvement, despite the entire course of three days. My symptoms got even worse.

Extreme body ache, very high fever, shivering, feeling cold and sore throat were my then symptoms. The symptoms were so bad that I never had such a severe illness before.

As I was hardly eating and hunger had almost disappeared, I could not, therefore, tell at that time if my sense of smell or taste had diminished.

I thought to myself that this is not a bacterial infection as antibiotics work for them. So it was bound to be a viral infection that does take a much longer time for recovery.

Whilst coming up the stairs, I was breathless and had to stop every three or four steps panting and gathering energy to move further.

The symptoms would sometimes aggravate and become quite extreme, and sometimes it would reduce by about 25% -35%, giving me some relief. After the three day course of antibiotics, another two days passed with very severe illness.

I had not showered or properly eaten for four or five days by that time. I was determined to persevere with the nibbling of snacks and medication.

For a person who regularly takes a shower at least once a day and if going to the gym then twice a day, not having a shower for days was not a comfortable experience.

However, I used disposable body wipes to clean and wipe off my body daily as I had no energy to step into the bath for a shower. The body aches simply did not let me get off the bed, and I mainly was sleeping for about 15 hours a day, but with no signs of recovery. This further compromised my regular eating.

The severity of illness continued to be on and off. Sometimes, the severity of the body aches, fever and shivering were quite substantial and next to unbearable. A few hours later, it used to be bearable enough for me to grab a small bite and have my paracetamol or ibuprofen dosage.

Discovery of the herb that did wonders

Given the days passing by and my body showing no signs of improvement, I had run out of all options so far as medication was concerned.

I had an urge to take a shower, hoping that it may bring some freshness and the water neutralize the negative energy in me. I decided to take a bath instead by simply lying in the bathtub filled with hot water, as taking a shower was just not possible for me due to my poor state.

The other reason I wanted to take a bath was that I

was feeling extremely cold despite the central heating on and the additional portable heater in the bedroom switched on as well. I thought that lying down in a hot bathtub might be comforting and provide some heat with the least possible effort.

I dragged myself to the bathroom, opened the bath tap and closed the plughole. With the hot water running and knowing that my body was aching badly, I decided to add some pink Himalayan salt hoping that it would soothe my aching body and provide some healing minerals for nourishment.

I dragged myself to the kitchen downstairs to grab the big Himalayan pink salt bag in this hope. Struggling my way up, I finally reached back to the bath.

I put about one full cereal bowl worth of Himalayan pink salt in the bathtub. Whilst putting in the salt, I thought I would not have the energy to use soap gel to clean myself thoroughly. I was also craving some freshness and needed something strong to cleanse my body.

I knew that tea tree essential oil is quite strong and has anti-viral and anti-microbial properties. I thought that tea tree oil seems like an excellent addition to the bath, given its anti-viral and anti-microbial properties. I had it handy in my walk-in wardrobe, which was close to the bathroom. I got the tea tree essential oil and put about 30-40 drops in the bath already filled with hot salt water. The smell of the tea tree oil was extremely strong, and I quickly took off my clothes and got into the bathtub.

I just stayed there in the bath for about one hour as it was very comforting.

The first 15-20 minutes, I just was almost lost in the bath given the extreme condition I was encountering. I was a bit concerned as well as to not drown after getting unconscious. As I am reasonably tall, I tried to sit in such a way that in case I fell unconscious, I do not drown.

Slowly and steadily, I started to feel a bit of ease. I

then started to be more aware of my surroundings. That would be about 15-25 minutes being inside the bath by then.

I then started to feel the steam being inhaled by me and could smell the tea tree oil in the steam. Inhaling the vapour with tea tree oil began to be quite comforting and soothing. Another 15-20 minutes in the bathtub, and I could start feeling the heat of the hot water in the bathtub more than before.

I then started feeling the body ache and headache diminishing rapidly, my head feeling light and me feeling much better.

Within an hour of being in the bathtub, I'd say my symptoms were reduced from 100% to about 15%-25%.

I came out of the bath after spending about an hour in it. I was feeling quite good, although I was exhausted by the effort made. I dried myself, wore fresh clothes and went straight to bed.

I was just in a state as if I have had the proper treatment and had started to heal. I felt at ease and very comforted. I lay down in bed. I slept for a very long time; I would say about 14 or 16 hours.

My journey back to normality

When I got up after the long sleep, I felt that my illness had almost gone. I would say it was reduced down to about 5% or even less. That does not mean that I was not feeling weak. I was feeling weak due to lack of eating yet energized at the same time to get moving. The body ache, the fever, the heaviness in the head, sore throat, headache etc., all just seemed to have vanished, giving me a sense of freedom and renewed life.

I was pretty elated and thanked the divine. I went downstairs to the kitchen and had something sufficient to eat. I knew that I had now recovered from the viral infection and was at the stage of a speedy recovery.

It is not uncommon for people who have a fever to

eat less during severe fever. In my case, it is the same, but when I recover, I tend to eat a bit more to replenish my body and, in particular, my muscles and return to my normal weight.

I am 5 feet 11 inches in height, and my weight was about 97 kilograms in the last week of December 2019. When I stood on the scales by the end of December 2019, my weight, after the end of my illness, had dropped to 90 kilograms.

It was a 7-kilogram drop in weight within a span of 1 week.

By the time I had recovered, it was only a day or two left for the new year, and then the offices re-opened. I went to the office and found out that two of my colleagues were severely ill, which is usually very uncommon during the new year period.

Within a few weeks after that, I started hearing about Covid 19 and its symptoms. When I heard about it, I was sure I had Covid 19 in December 2019.

When this news began to spread in the United

Kingdom, it was understood that Covid came to Britain at or around the end of January or February 2020.

Many did not believe it when I told them I already had the virus in December 2019. It was so severe I had never experienced anything like that ever before.

At the time, the media and the scientific community were pretty much consistent in reporting that the virus got in the United Kingdom around January or February 2020. Such news was not compatible with my gut feeling and my experience, but there was nothing I could do about it.

Oddly enough, I met a few people in February and March 2020 who said the same thing as I said that the illness they had at the end of December 2019 was something they had never experienced before. They all suspected to have been infected by Covid 19 in December 2019. They all had similar symptoms to the ones I had experienced and were identical to the ones the scientists were saying in or around February or March 2020 to be the symptoms of Covid 19. Like me, they all were confident that they had the virus in December 2019.

I was sure what I had was not a bacterial infection because I took antibiotics, which had no effect on the infection. It was only in later months in the year 2020 when it was accepted that Covid 19 was in the United Kingdom in 2019 and not the beginning of 2020.

That was my first infection with Covid 19, although not medically verifiable, given the then scarce information within the scientific community about it. Notwithstanding, one thing was for sure that tea tree oil was the herb that did wonders.

In the later chapters, I describe how I re-verified that tea tree oil does work for Covid 19 and is, in fact, in my view is the wonder herb for dealing with Covid 19.

CHAPTER 5

Defeating Covid 19 again

My second Covid infection happened in about mid-March or April 2020. It was a time when in the United Kingdom, talks about lockdown had begun. At that time, there were talks about people getting immune to this new virus, and it was hoped that once they have had the infection, they will not have it again for a long time. There were even talks about herd immunity, and everything was subject to deliberation.

I was following the news like everyone else quite thoroughly to see the developments that were happening, which were relatively rapid. Then in end-March or early April, I started to feel that I was coming down with something. It was like a feeling one gets before fever, and it was similar to the fatigue like feeling like I had experienced in December 2019.

However, this was just the start of getting this feeling. There were no body aches but mainly a headache-like feeling with a sense of being run-down, which people usually get before fever.

Given that the new virus was now well known to be in the United Kingdom, I had my suspicion that I had got the virus again, as I was going to the office every day due to work.

At that time, the news and media reported that persistent cough and high fever are the two main signs of the new virus. Being asymptomatic or losing the sense of smell or taste was not a symptom even discussed by anyone at that stage. What was then known about the virus was that it first attacked the lungs.

It was my third day of feeling low and Covid tests were not available to the public. Given that it was known for sure that Covid 19 is a virus that clings to the lung, I knew what to do.

It was late evening, and I had come back home from work. I took the tea tree oil bottle in my hand as tea tree oil is known to have anti-viral and anti-microbial properties. I opened the cap, brought the bottle closer to my nose and took deep breaths inhaling the tea tree oil directly from the bottle. The smell was quite strong. I inhaled it from one nostril by closing the other nostril with my fingers. I held my breath for a few seconds and then exhaled through the mouth and then repeated it a few times. I then inhaled from the same nostril, paused my breath to let the strong smell be in my lungs for a while before exhaling it through the other nostril closing the nostril with my hand from which I inhaled.

I did that for the other side of my nostril and repeated this process a few times. I would say about five or six times.

At the same time, after inhaling the wonder herb, I also took an Iodine supplement in an ionic form. I took only four drops orally, which is 500 mcg in total strength.

Iodine has also got anti-viral properties. It was night time when I did this, and the next day I got up for work as usual, very fresh and full of energy. The run-down feeling had gone entirely, and I was feeling very energized.

I took a shower and started getting ready for work. Once I was ready, I sprayed my cologne first on my clothes and then on my wrists, rubbing them against each other. Funnily I could not smell anything which was quite weird.

I sprayed a bit more on my wrist (the same cologne) and tried to smell the fragrance, but again I could not smell anything at all.

I smelled directly from the nozzle of the cologne bottle and could not smell anything as well. I thought for a second that the cologne, for some reason, had gone off as my sense of smell in general terms is extremely strong and much more developed in comparison to other peoples' ability to smell. Therefore it was not something that came to my immediate mind that losing my smell suddenly out of the blue was possible.

I tried another cologne of a different brand on my wrist, but I could not smell it either. I then tried a third bottle of my expensive perfume and could not smell it either.

Astounded, I went to my wife and asked her if she could smell any perfume on me, and I forwarded my wrist towards her nose. She said, "*oh, yes*". She said she could smell it very well, and it was pretty nice.

I found that extremely weird that my sense of smell had just gone as it was quite good even the night before when I snorted on the tea tree essential oil.

At the time, there was no news whatsoever about people losing the sense of smell due to the virus being reasonably new. I, therefore, could not have imagined that the loss of smell was due to Covid 19 infection.

Consequentially, I thought to myself that I have just got up and got ready, and it may be possible that my body hasn't fully started to function, or some nerve may have been pressed and numbed during sleep. Therefore, I decided to go to work thinking that walking and moving around would help and, if any nerve was pressed that caused the loss of smell, it might start to function as normal.

I reached the office without any concern as I had hoped that my sense of smell should be coming back within a few hours, given that I felt terrific health-wise.

When I reached the office at about 9:00 am, which is my usual time to start work, I spent about an hour working on my files and taking telephone calls. At about 10:00 am, I decided to have my usual cup of espresso.

My colleague kindly made me a cup of espresso and

brought it to me. I smelled it hoping that by then, I should have gotten my sense of smell back.

To my surprise, I could not smell anything at all despite an espresso ought to be having a powerful smell.

At this point, I decided to get myself checked and soon called my General Practitioner at my local medical centre near my house, where I had been registered.

I booked an appointment, and I confirmed while booking that I had no known symptoms of the new virus, which were then reported to be coughing, or persistent coughing and high fever. I went to the medical centre to see the doctor.

Having arrived at the medical centre, I waited for about 10 minutes before I was called in to see the doctor. The lady doctor checked my blood pressure asked me some basic questions about my health. I did not have any previous medical condition and so the only health issue I told her at that time was the loss of sense of smell; otherwise, I was in perfectly good health with no other symptom to complain about.

I also mentioned to the doctor that I have never lost my sense of smell before, and my sense of smell is quite good and generally much better than other people. The lady doctor was amazed that I was not displaying any other symptoms.

She checked my temperature and then did something on the computer and asked me a few more questions. She then made me do some movements to see if I was otherwise okay. I must say the doctor was quite impressive and very thorough in trying to diagnose my illness.

She then went out to take a second opinion and came back. When she came back after the second opinion, her smiling face was not to be seen. She now looked worrisome.

The doctor's sudden change of facial expression and body language were puzzling but did not scare me as I felt pretty good otherwise.

She said that losing the sense of smell was a sign of stroke, and I needed to rush straight to the hospital, and I should not even drive.

A stroke is a serious life-threatening condition when the blood supply has partly cut off from the brain, and sense of smell could be affected as a consequence.

She then picked up the phone and called the hospital to say that they need to make urgent arrangements to admit me. She gave my number to them over the phone.

After she hung up, she told me that I should go home and expect a call to go to the hospital. She said that depending upon which hospital has got availability, they would direct me to that one.

I asked her if I could drive, and she advised me strongly against it. I then left the medical centre and reached home within 10 minutes.

I just sat down for two minutes at home thinking about what I could eat for lunch when all of a sudden my mobile phone rang.

I picked up the phone and was told that it is from the hospital and I need to rush immediately without any delay to the hospital. I was strongly advised not to drive. I immediately called for a cab. The cab came reasonably quickly, and when I sat in, I asked the driver to take me to the City Hospital. He asked which section of the hospital he should drop me off, and I said A&E.

The driver was quite a pleasant and jolly chap, so he inquired if everything was okay or any of my family member was unwell. I responded to him, telling him that the doctor thinks I'm having a stroke, and so I am going to the A&E to get admitted. The driver just gave me a blank look. His facial expression told me that he did not know whether to console me or tell me everything will be okay or pray for me. The rest of the journey to the hospital was hence in silence.

At reaching the hospital, I was admitted in no time for checkups. I got my blood drawn for tests, blood pressure measured, ECG done and finally followed by a CT scan. Luckily, all results came out well.

At the end of nearly 11 hours at the hospital, when the CT scans finally gave an all-clear, the specialist doctor, possibly the hospital's radiologist, rechecked me. He made me do specific movements and noticed that I did not have slurred speech.

Finally, he told me to close my eyes and asked me to tell him if I could smell anything. I could not smell anything and told him accordingly. When I opened my eyes, it was digestive cookies that he had put close to my nose. The doctor said that the good thing is that it was not a stroke and told me to go home and make an appointment after two weeks with my general practitioner again for further diagnosis.

As it later transpired, I did not need another appointment with the doctor as my sense of smell came back in a few days by itself.

About a week or ten days later from this hospital incident, a random news article mentioned that many people had reported a loss of sense of smell due to Covid 19. That was the first news article I had seen or heard about the loss of smell being reported as a symptom of Covid 19. It was not a reliable news article, and so I could not rely on it for credibility.

Within a week or two after that, reliable media sources also mentioned that many people encountered a loss of smell due to the new virus.

Interestingly, when the first infection happened in December 2019, there was no news of the new virus in the United Kingdom. It was only later that it became officially apparent that Covid 19 was in Britain at the end of 2019.

Similarly, when my second infection happened in March or April 2020, there was talk of herd immunity and chances of being re-infected to be negligible. It was only a few months afterwards that it became clear that people can contract the new virus within a few months once again as the antibodies diminished reasonably quickly. Loss of smell as a symptom also got established later, and not when I had the infection.

My observation on both such instances demonstrated that ancient wisdom and gut feeling make a massive difference in life rather than exclusively relying on statistics and modern science. The latter has immense benefits but giving it entire credit in dealing with health issues is not appropriate.

The power of nature and human intuition cannot be underestimated. Even animals in the forest know what herbs to eat for getting better. When the tsunami happened, not only animals but humans who followed stone age cultures survived. Such cultures retained something that seemed lost in today's world. It is the connection with nature.

Modern science has no doubt hugely contributed to

the betterment of humanity, including health and well-being. But we cannot ignore the fact that the human body is part of mother nature, and so to find a solution in nature makes perfectly logical sense.

One thing was for sure that using tea tree oil did have an impact. On this second infection, I could smell the tea tree essential oil when I felt run down. I got better after smelling its strong scent, but the sense of smell by then had gone. I can only conclude by my experience that the strong smell of the tea tree oil is not taken nicely by the Covid 19 virus. It either deactivates the virus or attacks it. In doing so, it does seem to control the virus from spreading in the body further.

In the next chapter, I discuss how I already knew that the smell of tea tree oil has a powerful impact. The impact from the smell of tea tree oil was applied and tested by me in the past in general terms, and its results were astonishing.

This past knowledge of the power in the strong

scent of tea tree essential oil came in handy when applied for the new problem, i.e. Covid 19.

CHAPTER 6

The wonder herb discussed

The wonder herb that had a positive impact in dealing with my Covid 19 infection is tea tree essential oil. Tea tree essential oil is well known to be anti-bacterial, anti-fungal, anti-inflammatory and also anti-microbial.

Given the properties of tea tree essential oil, I have always had it in my house and have used it as a natural anti-fungal and anti-bacterial remedy primarily for skin conditions.

Tea tree essential oil is quite strong, and so the application of it on the skin can irritate the skin if one has got sensitive skin or if the skin condition is not normal. It is also often mixed with a carrier oil, such as olive oil, sesame seed oil etc., to make it more absorbable by the skin.

One must be extremely careful and aware that tea tree essential oil is never to be ingested, i.e. taken orally, as it is poisonous on consumption. It can be applied to the skin or inhaled but never consumed under any circumstances.

The power of tea tree essential oil

It is surprising how powerful this herb is. It is sometimes even stronger than the harsh chemicals available to deal with similar situations.

The first time I used tea tree oil was not for health reasons. About eight years ago, I was trying to find some remedy for a very thin line of mould (also spelt "mold") that had grown between the bay windows of my bedroom.

It was a minor mould issue, and because it was between the two windows, it was tough to get rid of it. I had heard that putting bleach and leaving it for a few hours gets rid of the mould. But on that occasion, it simply did not seem to work. So I did a bit of DIY research on the Internet where many different sprays were recommended, and then there was someone commenting on how tea tree oil diluted in water and sprayed on the mould can help with such issues.

As extremely powerful bleach had failed, I did want to get any more harsh chemicals as the smell of such harsh chemicals is considered quite harmful.

I had some tea tree oil in the house as part of a set of essential oils used with a diffuser. I put some of it in a spray bottle, probably about 10-15 drops with an inch of water in a small 250 ml spray bottle to spray on the mould that was within the corner line of the two bay windows. I sprayed over it and left it overnight, and the next day the mould had significantly reduced, in fact, almost disappeared with a little bit of trace.

I was pretty impressed that where bleach failed to do the job, tea tree oil which is just an essential oil, had worked. Also, tea tree oil was a natural alternative used instead of the very heavy chemical sprays that are so strong that they could be dangerous to health.

Although I read quite extensively over health products and natural-based supplements, tea tree oil had never previously been looked up by me. That was because it is not a supplement, i.e. it is not for oral consumption. To add to it, it is in fact, poisonous if taken orally.

This natural product had worked so well for the mould issue that it caught my attention. I soon started researching more about tea tree oil benefits as my interest had grown substantially. I learnt about its anti-bacterial, anti-inflammatory and anti-viral properties and started using it with success.

I started using it more in skin products and adding the tea tree essential oil to my face and body moisturizer for anti-bacterial and anti-fungal benefits. It worked pretty well, and adding tea tree oil did improve my skin condition generally. I accordingly became a regular user of it for skin health.

My other previous experiment that demonstrated the powerful effects of the tea tree's scent was to do with my sports shoes. Yes, that is right, my sports shoes!

I usually wear special five finger shoes when weight training at the gym. It is quite a unique shoe as it is meant to replicate barefoot feel and experience. It is like a foot glove for the feet but with a thin rubber layering underneath the sole for protection from tiny sharp objects when walking on the road or outdoors.

The socks worn with these shoes are also unique because they fit like a glove.

I found the socks quite uncomfortable as it was a bit tight on my toes. So I wear five finger shoes without any socks.

As you can imagine, weight training in shoes without

socks can, in a few weeks, cause the shoes to smell of foul odour.

I generally have good feet hygiene, and I am lucky not to have smelly feet. Even if I wear my socks during office hours with my work shoes, my work shoes and socks do not smell.

However, when training with my five finger shoes without socks, like any other sports shoes, would have, they do tend to smell with time. I used to wash the shoes in the washing machine with detergent, but a faint light smell of sweat just didn't seem to go even after washing them.

I started using special shoe sprays to eliminate the odour inside the shoes. While it did help, the smell was simply overpowering the foul odour with a stronger smell rather than eliminating the bad odour. It was not leaving the shoes smelling clean but instead smelling of the strong smell of the chemical used to overpower the existing odour.

As I was not satisfied with the hygiene, I then started

leaving the sports shoes immersed in water for some time and then brushing them with a cleaning brush before putting them in the washing machine and washing it with detergent.

Even then, there was a little bit of a smell in the shoes. I thought of putting some diluted bleach in the shoes before washing them to take care of the foul odour. However, bleach damages the fabric if the fabric is kept in for long as it is quite strong. Additionally, using bleach on fabric that will touch the body is not a good idea as it will irritate the skin.

Therefore, as an alternative, I thought of tea tree oil's strong scent and knowing its anti-bacterial, anti-fungal and anti-microbial properties, I decided to use it to try to get rid of the smell from my sports shoes.

So on the next occasion, when the shoes started to smell a bit more than the subtle smell remaining after washing, I decided to put a few drops of tea tree essential oil inside the shoes and leave it overnight. I had decided I would give it a nice wash the following day.

The following day, I was packing my gym bag, and I grabbed the shoes to put them in my gym bag with the intention that I would wash them in the evening. But when I smelled them before putting them in the bag, I was surprised that the foul odour and sweaty smell had completely gone. The shoes smelled so clean and fresh that they did not require washing anymore. The use of tea tree oil and its powerful smell had again proven to be far more effective than chemicals.

My experience of playing with this herb had helped me understand the significant impact the smell of this herb has on unwanted micro-organism overgrowth.

I even use a few tea tee oil drops with the washing detergent when washing clothes in the washing machine. I found that when using tea tree essential oil if the damp clothes were not taken out of the washing machine for hours after a wash, they still came out smelling fresh.

I, therefore, had enough experience of tea tree essential oil's benefits to deal with unwanted microbial growth.

Using the wonder herb for Covid-19

During my first Covid 19 infection in December 2019, I had put tea tree essential oil in the bathtub. The steam with this strong scent had a significant and almost immediate impact in dealing with my illness, from which I recovered almost fully the following day.

My use of tea tree oil on this first occasion for dealing with the new virus infection was conjectural in approach. One can call it a sheer accident through which I realized that the herb works for Covid 19. How ever one may view it, it no doubt worked miraculously for me.

On the second occasion of the Covid 19 infection, it was common ground that the virus first affects the lungs and settles there and then starts to cause a problem.

On the second occasion, which was at the end of March or April 2020, I suspected getting the virus again when I started to feel slightly low and similar to my first infection in December 2019. At that time, I already knew that tea tree oil had worked on a previous occasion, and I also knew that tea tree oil's scent is potent in dealing with unwanted micro-organisms.

I believed that if the new virus has entered my lungs, the best way to deal with it is to smell tea tree essential oil and hold my breath so that the strong scent inhaled deactivates or weakens the virus. I knew that inhaling tea tree oil was not dangerous to try as tea tree essential oil is otherwise available to be used in a diffuser to create a pleasant smell in the room. If breathing the nice scent in the room was considered good, then inhaling the oil could not intrinsically be bad.

I was not surprised that it did work again. When I inhaled the tea tree oil directly from the bottle, I found the smell very powerful. But the following day, my sense of smell had gone, although my run-down feeling had completely gone. I, therefore, consider that tea tree oil may either kill the virus or make it inactive or make it weak to such an extent that it starts to lose its hold over the body.

Shortly after my second Covid infection happened, my wife started to develop symptoms of sore throat and feverishness. My two-year-old daughter was also down with a slight fever. I used 30-40 drops of tea tree essential oil in the diffuser, and my wife's headache went within a few minutes, and she became energetic. She could work the entire day without any more feverish feeling or headache. Even my daughter recovered reasonably quickly.

My wife did not like the tea tree oil's smell on previous occasions when I used it with my body moisturizer. But on this occasion in 2020, she surprisingly said that she liked the smell. It was likely because it helped her soothe her symptoms and gave her a feeling of relaxation that made her start to enjoy the scent, as it is quite therapeutic.

I was pretty confident by then that tea tree oil seems to work against Covid 19. I was amazed that such a simple thing had not yet been researched or discovered by the scientific community. That can be understood as the scientific community had been overwhelmed with this new virus and looked at various other options to tackle the virus.

It has been a race in time to find a solution. Tea tree oil as a possible remedy to fight the virus appears to have gone unnoticed.

CHAPTER 7

Amazing results re-confirmed

After having tried tea tree essential oil on myself and my wife with positive results, it was time to offer it to others who had tested positive for Covid 19.

Many people are sceptical about trying herbal remedies, and this new virus is not common for people to have. Even if you know someone who has been tested positive, they may not be open to trying a herbal remedy. Also, by the time one finds out that someone has been tested positive, they may already have recovered.

There are quite a few who consider that when serious illnesses happen, then herbal remedies are ineffective. Therefore, it was tough to find someone I closely knew who was tested positive for Covid 19.

However, in November 2020, when I got to know that my former colleague had tested positive for Covid 19 along with her husband, I thought I should try and help them if they were willing to try the herb.

I telephoned my former colleague to check on her first. She said that she was having headaches, fever and was unable to bear the symptoms. The husband had severe body ache, but his condition was on and off. One could tell from her voice that she was in agony and distress.

I told her about this oil and how it had helped my wife and me. Given her debilitating condition, she was eager to try anything. Luckily my former colleague lived only two to three minutes' drive away from my house. Besides dropping some cooked food, I also separately kept the bottle of tea tree essential oil at her entrance door for her to collect.

After dropping the tea tree essential oil at my former colleague's house, I spoke to her and explained how to use it. Within an hour of such a telephone call, I got a text from her stating: *"thank you for the oil... my headache nearly gone... quite strong but feeling little better not 100% but will be okay... Thank you for all the help X"*.

When I later spoke to her during the day after the text, she mentioned that the tea tree oil had a considerable positive impact on her symptoms.

A few weeks later, when I spoke to her again, she said that her experience with tea tree oil has simply been "*amazing*".

Even in February 2021, when I asked her again to describe how much effective the tea tree oil was as I intended to write a book on it, she said it was amazing and said she was not exaggerating this. She even said that one of her friend and her husband had lately been tested positive for Covid 19, and she had given tea tree oil to them, and even they have had very positive feedback and could not thank enough. She also said that tea tree oil seemed to work when no medication worked. That was similar to my experience in dealing with Covid 19.

Therefore, I am confident that tea tree oil does have a significant impact on dealing with Covid 19. Of course, every individual is different and responds differently. That said, I see no reason why this herb would not make a difference in the lives of people who may get infected with Covid 19 and display symptoms.

That is in no way to dissuade people from getting vaccinated. By the time people get an opportunity to be vaccinated, there will be many hundreds and thousands of people who may get infected by the virus. They would have to deal with the illness without the benefit of the vaccine. Even if people get inoculated, the chances of getting severe symptoms are said to be reduced but not eliminated.

With the new strains, one also does not know where the future lies and how effective and long the vaccine will give adequate protection.

Tea tree oil has shown very positive results in my experience. I hope that it will benefit all persons who, in the unlikely event, get infected with Covid 19 and show symptoms from mild to severe.

Please also note that one should not ignore medical advice and not hesitate to contact the medical practitioner. Please also follow the guidelines set by the relevant country you are in.

CHAPTER 8

Proper administration of the herb

It is very important to understand how to use tea tree essential oil for optimum results. It's the strong scent emitted by the oil when inhaled that seems to help attack the virus by either making it inactive or weakening its hold on the body.

If one has no energy to do anything because of the severity of symptoms due to Covid 19, they can smell the tea tree oil straight from the bottle by bringing the bottle close to their nose. In doing so, inhale from one nostril while closing the other nostril with a finger. Hold the breath for a second or two and exhale from the other nostril closing the one from which you initially inhaled. Repeat this process from both nostrils.

One can also take two or three drops of the tea tree essential oil and rub it inside both the nostrils so that there is continued inhalation of the oil. Tea tree oil is quite strong and can have a burning effect if one has got sensitive skin. So try very little if not sure first.

If the inside of the nostrils is too sensitive for the tea tree oil application, then dab some outside the nostrils, i.e. above the lips.

One can also put a few drops of tea tree oil on a handkerchief and keep smelling the cloth for inhaling the strong scent of the oil.

In my view, however, it would be best to inhale the steam containing water with 10 to 15 drops of tea tree oil. This way, the steam will carry the water droplets with the tea tree oil in a similar fashion to the virus that got into the system. Inhaling the vapour will be easier for the body to get the full effects of tea tree oil's anti-viral and anti-microbial scent.

Steaming can be done by taking a small bowl filled with hot water and adding 10 to 15 drops in it or more, as long as the smell is not too strong to bear.

As stated in previous chapters, no matter what happens, do not ingest tea tree oil as it is poisonous when ingested. If one has a humidifier, then put 20 to 40 drops in water, and the humidifier will make the atmosphere not only soothing but will also help in continuous inhalation of tea tree oil without much effort.

The proof lies in the pudding. My wife and I, my former colleague, and her friends are living examples of how this wonder herb has benefited us in dealing with Covid 19.

Tea tree essential oil is an inexpensive herb, and one only needs a small bottle of 5 ml or 10 ml to do the trick.

This gift of mother nature has been a blessing, and I hope all can benefit from this home remedy.

One should not expect to succeed without trying.

Let it be a fight against Covid 19 or anything else in life. If we close our avenues, then our options get automatically limited.

We should never underestimate the power of nature, no matter how advanced modern science may take us. We are humans, and as humans, we are physically subject to the laws of nature. The laws of nature are to help humanity evolve and prosper, not deteriorate. Harnessing the power of nature, therefore, is the key to health and well-being.

CHAPTER 9

Covid and mental health

Many people have had a challenging time during this pandemic, with a lot of uncertainty in businesses, industries and jobs. Lockdown has also taken away our freedom.

Many jobs have been lost, and many jobs have been put under scrutiny. Many people have been unable to pay mortgages, and many have not been able to pay their rent.

Apart from financial difficulties during this pandemic that has created stress in our lives, we see students, elderly living away from their loved ones, young children, doctors, nurses, working professionals and many others put under difficult situation.

A problematic situation takes a toll on mental health if one does not take a constructive step in relaxing the mind. A relaxed mind can take in far more pressures with ease in comparison to an overworked mind.

Many people feel that taking in stress is a part of everyday life, and for the tension to go away with time is considered normal.

Some take on healthy dietary habits to reduce the level of stress.

Physical activity especially exercises that lead to physical exertion, but not extreme physical exertion does help to reduce stress levels. It is a literal way to throw the negative energy out of our system, which then gets neutralized by mother nature.

One must realize that we feel unhappy or stressed when things do not go as expected. Consequentially, the unwanted circumstances create a problem for the mind to resolve. It is a burden added on the mind, and the mind is put to its natural task to solve the problem.

This problem is what we call mind related stress. If not resolved by the mind or how much significance the mind gives to such a situation impacts the mind's health. In the long run, this throws the mind off balance and causes mental health issues.

The body affects the mind and vice-versa. Therefore, keeping a healthy and well-nourished body should not be ignored when dealing with mental health.

Furthermore, a realization needs to set in that the human body does not care about how much wealth one has acquired in its natural state. The human body does not care about how many houses or properties one may have acquired. The human body does not care about how successful one's business is. The human body does not care about how famous one may be. The importance we give to worldly things is just how the mind has been trained by observing the environment it has been exposed to.

All these things concerning wealth and societal successes should not affect the mind as it does not affect the human body, which includes the mind. But because we generally focus mainly on the areas concerning financial matters, family, success, body, food, beauty, fame etc., the mind starts to dwell on these areas. It dwells to such great extent that it finds it at times inseverable to such things we focus upon. In this process, it starts to feel accustomed and attached to these material things, and any event that takes such a thing away or a perceived threat of it going away causes the mind to feel the pain and stress of separation or loss.

At other times, the mind also feels that it has failed to fix the problem. That is the unnecessary stress we create and is not needed. All such material things the mind focuses upon are only good so long as it does not adversely affect the mind or our health.

Invest some time for the mind

There is no doubt that for a healthy mind, a healthy body is essential. But it is also vital that the mind has its own specific time devoted to relaxation. It needs to take a break from thinking and from focusing on worldly things and issues all the time. Only then can it work at its optimum and not affect the health adversely.

Physical exercise does, to some extent, help the mind to take a break. But physical activity is not directly targeting the mind as such. The exercise which is directly beneficial to the mind is the exercise of meditation.

Yes, meditation is an exercise (or in other words activity) for the mind, and if done correctly, it makes the mind work better, healthier and more robust.

Meditation is not about sitting in a spot and doing nothing. That would not be an exercise then. Meditation involves the active participation of the mind.

There are many techniques for meditation at the beginner level. The ultimate aim for all such methods is to still the mind, i.e. having no thoughts. It is not being absent-minded or being idle as that would not be an exercise that requires active participation by the mind.

Although there are hundreds of meditation techniques, the starting aim is to let the mind focus on one thing only. In doing so, the thoughts during the meditation sitting start to decrease, which provides relaxation to the mind. That is because the more the mind thinks, the more exhausted it gets.

Mind's job is to think. So for the mind to take a break and relax, it needs not to think. When the mind continues to think without a break, several thoughts go on within the mind. With time and with numerosity of thoughts comes chaos resulting in agitation and confusion. Meditation helps to disentangle the thoughts and ease the burden put on the mind.

Meditation helps us to still our mind so that eventually, there are no thoughts. This state of no-thought is an active state of mind and is different from a passive state of absent-mindedness.

Through the practice of meditation with time, unnecessary thoughts tend to decrease. As a result, the mind can better focus on things that matter. Accordingly, efficiency and productivity increases and the overall health of the mind improves.

Technique of meditation

Whilst there are many techniques for the practice of meditation that I have tried with success, I only discuss the method here, which is more suitable for mental health.

One can start this exercise of meditation by sitting in a relaxed place with no disturbance. If one has had a very troublesome day or the mind is being very erratic, then before sitting, they can spend 2-5 minutes in any kind of physical exercise. It can be done in the same room where one is to sit so that one does not get distracted by the activity to such an extent that they decide not to sit for meditation. It could be simple push-ups or still jogging or anything that causes some physical exertion. For beginners, brief physical activity before the mediation sitting is beneficial but not necessary. As one progresses in meditation, the short physical activity before the meditation can be left out completely.

For meditation, any comfortable pose should be used. The idea is to be relaxed and not having any thought. An uncomfortable posture will keep on signalling the mind about the discomfort the body is experiencing. So, to begin with, choose a comfortable position. It could be sitting on a chair or sofa or anything where one can sit comfortably for a few minutes.

For the first five minutes, some soothing devotional music could be listened, if the mind is very much at unrest. That again is not necessary, but if one is to listen to music, try to be attentive to it with eyes closed when listening to such music. Also, try listening to instrumental or devotional music only as such music is generally not focused on worldly things that can take our minds in that direction again, as this would defeat the purpose of decreasing the thoughts.

Once the preliminaries are over and the eyes are closed, repeat in mind any word or combination of words that soothe the mind. The word (or the combination) could be love, peace, bliss, harmony, divine light or any name of God which one believes in. The chosen word or words should not be an expression of worldly things as that would distract the focus in the long run.

Ensure that this repetition is done slowly in mind with 1-2 second pause before the next repetition. Each such repetition should be done attentively in mind and with as much contemplation as possible.

This process can be done for 5 minutes to start with and increased to 20-30 minutes gradually.

There may be quite a few thoughts that may barge in during this practice. Just mentally acknowledge such thoughts quickly and continue with the repetition. The acknowledgement of the thought should be just like how we recognize in our mind a task that is to be done later once the present task we are doing is over.

As this is an exercise for the mind, one may initially feel the need to sleep longer and deeper during the early days of practice. That is a good sign to show that the mind did take an active part in the process.

After the longer and deeper sleep, one would feel mentally refreshed and, with time, more focused on reality than superficiality. This way, the mind will become a helping companion for the body rather than creating troubles of its own. That, in turn, increases our efficiency and productivity and helps us move towards a state of equipoise where our emotions are also well balanced.

In the context of mental health, meditation is a

practice of rebooting the mind so that it functions better. It is a cost-free way of retuning the mind for optimum health.

So meditate for a stress-free, happy and healthy life.

ABOUT THE AUTHOR

G Sambi is a lawyer by profession, a philosopher at heart, and a holistic healer by interest.

Since childhood, he has been interested in the undiscussed reality of life. Having completed his Masters of Law from London in 2005, he has been working full time as a lawyer based in England, UK. On the side, he devotes time to holistic healing, naturopathy, Korean acupuncture and meditation.

Fighting Covid Naturally

Printed in Great Britain
by Amazon